TREMORS
What Is Hand Tremor
Signs, Symptoms, and Treatment

Pierre Mouchette, author

Life-Health Media USA
An Enviro | Life Knowledge Publication
a subsidiary of Real Property Experts LLC

Copyright © 2022 by Pierre Mouchette

All rights reserved. No part of this publication may be reproduced, distributed, or transmitted in any form or by any means, including photocopying, recording, or other electronic or mechanical methods, without the prior written permission of the publisher, except in the case of brief quotations embodied in critical reviews and specific other noncommercial uses permitted by copyright law.

ISBN 979-8422647170 (Paperback Book)

Independently Published

First Edition: February 2022
Life-Health Media USA
Web Address: https://www.enviro-life-media.com
Contact: publications@synchronicity-investor.com

Note: This publication comes in various formats, such as Paperbacks and Electronic Books (e-books). Particular material in the paperback version of this book may not be included in e-books, and vice versa.

At Life-Health Media USA, we pride ourselves on every publication's quality, research, and transparency. All content is carefully researched.

Disclaimer:

This Life-Health Media USA publication provides information about the subject matter covered. The author and publisher of this content are not acting as healthcare professionals to present covered material. The information and statements are educational and not a substitute for informed medical advice. Do not take any action before consulting with a healthcare professional. You are exclusively responsible for the use of any content. You hold Life-Health Media USA and its members harmless in any event or claim, demand, or damage, including reasonable attorneys' fees, asserted by any third party, or arising out of your use of, or conduct on, publications and products.

Life-Health Media writers provide applicable content and break down complex topics so they are easier to understand. Information given may not apply to your specific situation, and products or services recommended may not be a good fit for your application. While Life-Health Media USA strives to provide accurate, up-to-date content, we cannot guarantee the accuracy and completeness of the information supplied. By using this content, you understand that all material is an expression of opinion and not professional advice.

The contents of this publication were developed through the writings of licensed and non-licensed medical professionals and other external contributors and are for informational purposes only. The content herein is not a substitute for professional medical advice, diagnosis, or treatment. Always consult your doctor or other qualified healthcare providers with any questions regarding a medical condition, procedure, or treatment. Whether a prescription medication, over-the-counter medicine, vitamin, supplement, or herbal alternative, your physician should review all drugs before purchase or use.

Life-Health Media USA makes no guarantees about the efficiency or safety of products or treatments described in its content. Health conditions and drug information are subject to change and do not include all applications, instructions, contraindications, drug interactions, allergic reactions, or adverse effects.

Life-Health Media USA does not recommend or endorse any specific test, clinician, clinical care provider, product, procedure, opinion, or service mentioned in Life-Health Media USA publications. This publication is not a substitute for informed medical advice, and you should not take any action before consulting with your healthcare provider.

WHAT ARE TREMORS

Tremors are an involuntary, rhythmic, oscillatory movement of a body part. This is also the most common movement disorder that affects the hands. Tremors may also occur in the arms, head, vocal cords, torso, and legs. They can happen sporadically, constantly, or due to a disorder. A tremor can be qualified as **enhanced physiologic, essential, and parkinsonian.**

In general, tremor is caused by a problem in the deep parts of the brain that control movements. Most tremors have no known cause, although some forms appear to be inherited (genetic) and run-in families.

Everyone has low-amplitude, high-frequency physiologic tremor at **rest** and during an **action** that is not symptomatic but is augmented by anxiety, medication use, caffeine intake, or fatigue.

Contents

SECTION 1　TREMORS ....- 9 -
  What Causes Tremor ....- 10 -
  How Are Tremors Diagnosed? ....- 11 -
  Describing Tremors ....- 12 -
  Types Of Tremors ....- 14 -
    Physiologic Tremor (PT) ....- 14 -
    Essential Tremor (ET) ....- 14 -
    Cerebellar and Rubral Tremor ....- 15 -
    Drug-Induced Tremor ....- 15 -
    Dystonic Tremor ....- 16 -
    Intention Tremor ....- 16 -
    Neuropathic Tremor ....- 17 -
    Orthostatic Tremor ....- 17 -
    Parkinsonian Tremor ....- 17 -
    Psychogenic Tremor ....- 18 -
  Metabolic Disorders ....- 19 -
  Available Tremor Treatments ....- 20 -
    Focused Ultrasound ....- 21 -
    Surgery ....- 21 -
  Dealing With Tremor ....- 23 -

SECTION 2　HAND TREMOR ....- 24 -
  What Is A Hand Tremor? ....- 26 -
  Tremor Descriptions ....- 26 -
  Neurological Conditions ....- 27 -
  Hand Tremor Conditions and Symptoms ....- 29 -

General Health Conditions .... - 29 -
Symptoms That Might Occur With Hand Tremor .... - 29 -
SECTION 3   CAUSES of HAND TREMOR .... - 31 -
Not Always a Disease .... - 32 -
Potential Causes Of Hand Tremor .... - 33 -
Potential Medications That Cause Tremor Symptoms ... - 33 -
Complications Of Hand Tremor..................................... - 35 -
Hand Tremor Triggers.. - 36 -
Diabetes.. - 41 -
Hypoglycemia .... - 41 -
Diabetic Neuropathy.. - 41 -
SECTION 4   TREATMENT .... - 42 -
Seeking Medical Help .... - 43 -
Questions The Doctor Will Ask..................................... - 43 -
Some Treatment Medications .... - 44 -
What Medications Treat Shaky Hands? .... - 44 -
Commonly Prescribed Medications............................... - 44 -
Therapies and Surgery .... - 46 -
Therapy .... - 46 -
Surgery... - 46 -
Lifestyle Changes .... - 48 -
Stop Hands From Shaking .... - 48 -
APPENDIX A - DISEASES, DISORDERS, & CONDITIONS - 51 -
Fragile X Tremor Ataxias Syndrome (FXTAS) .... - 52 -
Hyperthyroidism (overactive thyroid)............................... - 53 -
Multiple Sclerosis (MS).. - 53 -

Multiple System Atrophy (MSA) .... - 54 -
Neurodegenerative Disease .... - 54 -
Parkinson's Disease (PD) .... - 55 -
Pheochromocytoma .... - 56 -
Tardive Dyskinesia .... - 56 -
Wilson's Disease .... - 57 -

APPENDIX B - TREATMENTS & EQUIPMENT .... - 58 -
Deep Brain Stimulation (DBS) .... - 59 -
Focused Ultrasound Thalamotomy .... - 62 -
Magnetic Resonance Imaging (MRI) .... - 64 -
Nerve Conduction Study (NCS) .... - 66 -

APPENDIX C - RESOURCES .... - 67 -
Organizations .... - 68 -
Website Articles .... - 69 -

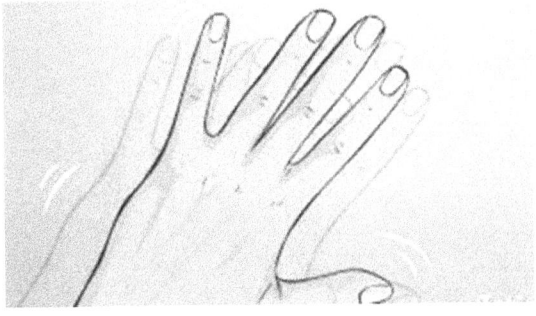

TREMORS - What Is Hand Tremor, Signs, Symptoms, and Treatment

SECTION 1   TREMORS

What Causes Tremor

A tremor can happen on its own or be a symptom associated with several neurological problems, that include:

- multiple sclerosis
- stroke
- traumatic brain injury
- neurodegenerative diseases affecting parts of the brain

Some other known causes include:

- alcohol abuse or withdrawal
- anxiety or panic.
- liver or kidney failure
- mercury poisoning
- overactive thyroid
- the use of certain medicines (some asthma medication, amphetamines, caffeine, corticosteroids, and drugs used for certain psychiatric and neurological disorders)

How Are Tremors Diagnosed?

Tremors are diagnosed through a physical and neurological examination and a thorough medical history review. During the physical evaluation, the doctor will evaluate the tremor based on the following:

- If the tremor happens when the muscles are at **rest** or in **action**
- Location of the tremor, and if it appears on one or both sides of the body
- The appearance of the tremor, its frequency, and amplitude

The doctor will check for other neurological findings such as impaired balance, speech abnormalities, and elevated muscle stiffness. A blood or urine test can rule out metabolic causes such as thyroid malfunction and certain medications that can cause tremor. These tests will also help identify contributing causes such as drug interactions, chronic alcoholism, and other conditions or diseases. Diagnostic imaging can help to determine if the tremor results from brain damage.

Additional tests may be required to determine functional limitations such as difficulty with handwriting or the ability to hold a fork or cup.

The doctor may also order an electromyogram to diagnose muscle or nerve troubles. The test measures involuntary muscle activity and muscle response to nerve stimulation.

Describing Tremors

Several terms are used to describe tremors, with the descriptions falling into two primary groups as follows:

Rest tremors - occur in a relaxed (static) body part that is entirely supported against gravity. Rest tremor is usually caused by **Parkinson's** but may also occur in severe **essential tremor.**

Action tremors - most tremors are **action tremors,** which occur with voluntary muscle contraction. Action tremors are subdivided into five different action subcategories.

- **Postural tremors** - is present while voluntarily maintaining a position against gravity. It includes **cerebellar, dystonic, essential, neurotic, physiologic,** and **drug-induced tremor.**

- **Intention tremor** - occurs with target-directed movements. The tremor typically worsens as a person draws closer to the target.

- **Isometric tremor** - occurs with muscle contraction against a rigid stationary object.

- **Kinetic tremors** - are associated with any form of voluntary movement. It includes **cerebellar, dystonic, and drug-induced tremor (essential tremors** can cross over to this category).
  - **Intention tremor** (a subtype) is produced with target-directed activities when the hand performs a voluntary action. The presence of this type of tremor implies that there is a disturbance of the cerebellum or its pathways.

Action tremors are based on the specific activity or tasks that trigger the tremor. Action tremor symptoms are characteristic of various diseases, disorders, and conditions, including essential tremor, drug withdrawal, stroke, brain tumor, and Multiple Sclerosis.

Types Of Tremors

Having a tremor classified correctly will help the healthcare professional provide the correct treatment for the condition. There are over twenty different types of tremors. Some common tremor types are:

Physiologic Tremor (PT)

Everyone has a physiologic tremor, even though it is not very noticeable. This is the tremor noticed when you hold your hand out with fingers extended. It may become more prominent (becoming an enhanced physiological tremor) due to anxiety, fatigue, using a stimulating substance like caffeine, fever, alcohol withdrawal, low blood sugar, some medications, and much more.

- **Enhanced physiological tremor** - a more noticeable case of physiologic tremor can be easily seen. A neurological disease does not cause it but a reaction to some drugs, alcohol withdrawal, medical conditions, including an overactive thyroid, and hypoglycemia. It goes away when the underlying cause is corrected. This tremor is not a disease and is not a concern.

Essential Tremor (ET)

This tremor is the most widespread of the many types of tremors. It is an **action tremor,** the most prominent kind of tremor. Since the tremor occurs when doing things, it can result in annoying problems such as spilling coffee and bringing food to the mouth with a utensil, writing, drawing, or typing and repeating the same character. The tremor usually shows up on both sides of the body but is more often noticed on the dominant hand because it is an **action tremor.**

This tremor can start at any age and progresses slowly. It usually increases with age, affecting people over 40. Essential tremor can be amplified by extreme emotion, stress, physical exhaustion, and low blood sugar.

*Note: research indicates that essential tremor may have a strong genetic component affecting multiple generations of families (It is referred to as **familial tremor**).*

Cerebellar and Rubral Tremor

The cerebellar tremor is an **intention tremor,** which is most noticeable in the act of coordination, such as pushing a button. Here, the tremor becomes more exaggerated as the finger is about to meet its target. This tremor is caused by brain damage to the cerebellum and its pathways to other brain regions resulting from a stroke, tumor, degenerative disease (Multiple Sclerosis), an inherited degenerative disorder such as ataxia (a loss of muscle control in the arms and legs), and Fragile X syndrome (a condition of intellectual and developmental problems). Chronic alcoholism can also cause **cerebellar tremor.**

- **Rubral tremor** is a rare cerebellar tremor subset. It is slow, significant in amplitude, and can occur in all directions. There are no simple treatments for cerebellar tremors.

Drug-Induced Tremor

There are a wide variety of medications that cause tremor. A drug-induced tremor is typically symmetric or equal on both sides of the body. It is a rhythmic, uncontrollable movement. Drug-induced tremor may also be described as **Drug-Induced Parkinson's (DIP).** If taking a new drug, be attentive to whether a tremor starts afterward. If it happens, discuss this with your doctor, and consult them before adding any new over-the-counter medications.

Note: anyone can develop tremor from taking medication. Still, some individuals are at greater risk than others. Those at increased risk are anyone with a history of dementia, people infected with HIV; the elderly; and women.

Dystonic Tremor

Dystonia is a movement disorder where incorrect messages from the brain cause muscle to be overactive, leading to abnormal postures or persistent unwanted (involuntary) movements. Dystonic tremor appears in young or middle-aged adults and can affect any muscle in the body.

This tremor may constitute an attempt to correct the unusual muscle contraction that repeatedly fails. In contrast to other forms of tremor, moving or holding the body in a specific fashion can worsen **dystonic tremor.** The tremor is likely to improve with rest or by touching parts of the body (usually but not always, the region affected by dystonia).

Intention Tremor

This tremor results when muscle contraction amplifies and the tremor increases as the individual enacts a deliberate and visually guided movement. As the individual moves with **intention,** the tremor occurs vertically and in the direction of the action, and the object aimed for is overshot. Intention tremors result from dysfunction or damage to the cerebellum or its pathways (i.e., a lesion, multiple sclerosis, or other degenerative or metabolic disorders).

Neuropathic Tremor

A tremor can be a sign of neuropathy, a disorder of the peripheral nerves. These are the nerves that bring messages from the brain and spinal cord to the rest of the body. Neuropathies triggered by autoimmune syndromes such as **Chronic Inflammatory Demyelinating Polyneuropathy (CIDP)** may have tremor as a component. A tremor in this situation is not an isolated symptom but is evaluated in the context of other signs of CIDP, which can include weakness, numbness, and tingling. Assessment by a neurologist can determine if the neuropathic tremor is a diagnostic consideration.

Neurodegenerative diseases like **parkinsonian syndromes Multiple System Atrophy (MSA)** can have tremors as a symptom. Other, more uncommon neurodegenerative diseases apart from **Parkinson's Disease (PD)** and typical parkinsonian syndromes can manifest tremor. Two of these include **Wilson's Disease** and **Fragile X Tremor Ataxia Syndrome (FXTAS)**. These diseases have complex symptomatology, and the larger neurologic picture aids in making the diagnosis.

Orthostatic Tremor

With this rare disorder, the legs and trunk start trembling soon after standing. Someone with **orthostatic tremor** might not notice a tremor so much as the unsteadiness after standing up. It improves soon after the affected sits down. The cause of orthostatic tremor is unknown.

Parkinsonian Tremor

Parkinsonian tremor is much more apparent when hands are at rest. But the legs, chin, and body may also be involved. Like any other tremor, Parkinsonian tremor can also be exacerbated by stress. Regardless of the name, Parkinsonian tremor is not always caused by Parkinson's disease, but may also be triggered by other neurodegenerative disorders, drugs, infections, and toxins. If Parkinson's disease causes the tremor, it usually starts more on one side of the body than the other.

Psychogenic Tremor

Like other psychogenic disorders, **psychogenic tremor** is a diagnosis of exclusion, which means other forms of tremor must be excluded. A psychogenic tremor is also referred to as a **functional tremor.** Clues that tremor is psychogenic include the fact that the tremor stops when distracted. The tremor suddenly recurs after a stressful incident, or frequent and otherwise unexplainable changes in the body part are affected by the tremor. Many people with psychogenic tremor have an underlying psychiatric disorder such as depression or **post-traumatic stress disorder (PTSD).**

Metabolic Disorders

Certain metabolic disturbances such as hyperthyroidism (or excessive thyroid hormone production) can lead to tremor. This condition may be distinguished from a pure tremor disorder by symptoms that accompany the tremor. These include weight loss, palpitations, excessive sweating, nervousness, and a tendency to be overheated. However, checking thyroid hormone levels will help identify this disorder in people with a new tremor.

Hypoglycemia or low glucose can similarly cause tremor. The hypoglycemia tremor is also typically accompanied by other symptoms, including sweating, dizziness, hunger, and irritability.

Available Tremor Treatments

Although there are no cures for most tremors, treatment options are available to help manage their symptoms. In some instances, a person's symptoms may be mild enough not to need treatment.

Finding a suitable treatment depends on an accurate diagnosis of the cause. The tremor caused by an underlying health problem can sometimes be improved or eliminated with treatment. For example, tremor resulting from thyroid hyperactivity will improve or even resolve (return to the normal state) with the treatment of the thyroid malfunction. If the tremor is caused by medication, stopping the tremor-causing drug can reduce or eliminate the tremor.

If there is no underlying cause for the tremor, it can be modified. Available treatment options include:

- Beta-blocking drugs such as propranolol are used to treat high blood pressure, but they also help treat **essential tremor.** Propranolol can also be used with other types of **action tremor.** Additional beta-blockers that can be used include atenolol, metoprolol, nadolol, and sotalol.

- Antiseizure medications such as primidone can be effective in people with **essential tremor** that do not respond to beta-blockers. Other prescribed drugs include gabapentin and topiramate. It is important to note that some antiseizure medications may cause tremor.

- Tranquilizers (also known as benzodiazepines) like alprazolam and clonazepam may **temporarily** help tremor. However, their use is limited by unwanted side effects, including sleepiness, poor concentration, and coordination. This may affect the ability of people to carry out everyday activities such as driving, school, and work. Furthermore, when taken regularly, tranquilizers can cause physical dependence and, when stopped abruptly, can cause various withdrawal effects.

- Parkinson's disease medications (levodopa, carbidopa) can be used to treat tremor linked to Parkinson's disease.

- Botulinum toxin can be used to treat almost all types of tremor. It is beneficial for head tremor, which does not respond to medications. Botulinum toxins are used to control **dystonic tremor.** Although botulinum toxin injections can decrease tremor for several months, they can also create muscle weaknesses. While this treatment is effective and is usually well tolerated for head tremor, botulinum toxin treatment in the hands can cause difficulties in fingers. It may also cause a hoarse voice and difficulty swallowing when treating voice tremor.

Focused Ultrasound

Treatments for **essential tremor** use **Magnetic Resonance Images (MRI)** to deliver focused ultrasound to create a lesion in the tiny areas of the brain's thalamus thought to be responsible for causing the tremor. The treatment is approved only for individuals with **essential tremor** who do not respond to anticonvulsant or beta-blocking drugs.

Surgery

If the patient does not respond to drug therapies or has a severe tremor, it significantly impacts their daily lives. In that case, their doctor may recommend surgical interventions such as **Deep Brain Stimulation (DBS)** or, very rarely, **Thalamotomy.**

While DBS is usually well-tolerated, tremor surgery's most common side effects are dysarthria (problems with speech) and balance difficulties.

- **Deep Brain Stimulation (DBS)** - is the most common surgical treatment for tremor. This method is preferred because it is practical, low risk, and treats a more extensive range of symptoms than thalamotomy. The treatment uses surgically implanted electrodes sending high-frequency electrical signals to the thalamus (the part of the brain which coordinates and controls involuntary movements). Here a tiny pulse generating device placed under the skin in the upper chest sends electrical stimuli to the brain, temporarily disabling a tremor. **DBS is used to treat parkinsonian tremor, essential tremor, and dystonia.**

- **Thalamotomy** - is a surgical procedure that requires the precise, permanent destruction of a tiny area in the thalamus. Surgery is replaced by radiofrequency ablation for treating severe tremor when deep brain surgery is contraindicated. Radiofrequency ablation utilizes a radio wave to generate an electrical current that heats up a nerve and disrupts its signaling ability, typically for six or more months. This procedure is performed on only one side of the brain to improve tremor on the opposite side of the body. Surgical procedure on both sides is not recommended as it can cause problems with speech.

Dealing With Tremor

Physical, speech-language, and occupational therapy may help control tremor and meet the challenges caused by the tremor. A physical therapist can help individuals improve their muscle control, functioning, and strength through coordination, balancing, and other exercises. Some therapists recommend using weights, splints, adaptive equipment, special plates, and utensils for eating. Speech-language pathologists assess and treat speech, language, communication, and swallowing disorders. Occupational therapists teach new ways to perform daily activities that tremors may affect.

Decreasing tremor-inducing substances such as caffeine and other medication (such as stimulants) can help improve tremor.

SECTION 2   HAND TREMOR

HAND TREMOR

Shaky hands are commonly known as a hand tremor. Having hand tremor is not life-threatening, but it can make performing everyday tasks problematic. This tremor could also be an early warning sign of neurological and degenerative disorders. The leading cause of shaking hands in adults is **essential tremor.** A condition doctors do not fully understand.

There are many possible causes for hand tremor, and you might be worried that your hand tremor indicates a more severe problem. In most cases, you should know that the cause of hand tremor usually is not serious. The condition is treatable and can be manageable in most occurrences.

This publication focuses on the **Quality of Life** of those affected by this disorder. Here we explain **'What Are Hand Tremor, Signs, Symptoms, and Treatment'** in an easy-to-read and understand format. The reader can utilize the information to help them understand the disorder more fully, relieve symptoms, understand treatments, and how their lifestyle affects them.

Information given will help the reader effectively reduce the conditions of this disorder, thereby enhancing their Quality of Life.

What Is A Hand Tremor?

It is an involuntary muscle movement consisting of trembling or shaking hands. Tremor most accurately refers to a slight, rhythmic shaking movement occurring in a back-and-forth pattern. However, everyone has an unnoticeable shaking when moving their hands. Fatigue, stress, anger or fear, caffeine, and smoking can make normal shaking more noticeable. Hand tremor can happen at any age but is common in middle-aged and older men and women.

Note: tremor primarily impacts the hands. However, tremor can also occur in other body parts, such as the head, the arms, the legs, the torso, and the voice box (larynx), which may cause a shaky voice.

Tremor Descriptions
Various Types

- **Post-stroke tremor** - following a stroke, one can get a variety of tremors. If there is damage to the cerebellum, this is an **intention tremor.** If damage is in the basal ganglia, the person can have a **resting tremor.**

- **Medication-induced tremor** - some medications can cause tremor, such as the antidepressant bupropion (Wellbutrin) and the anti-arrhythmic drug amiodarone (Cordarone). The resulting tremor is often **postural.**

- **Withdrawal tremor** - those suffering from alcohol withdrawal can experience **postural tremor.**

- **Essential tremor** - most widespread of the many types of tremors. The exact cause of this tremor is unknown, but a genetic component is involved in many cases, meaning that you can inherit essential tremor from your parents. Essential tremor can be amplified by extreme emotion, stress, physical exhaustion, and low blood sugar.

Short-term tremor that goes away quickly can be caused by an anxiety attack or stress, whereas chronic tremor that comes and goes over a more extended time can be due to essential tremor.

Even if it is temporary, all tremor need to be evaluated by a medical professional. Some hand tremor can be due to severe, ongoing diseases like Parkinson's and Multiple Sclerosis. Hand tremor from one side of the body could indicate damage to the brain from a tumor or stroke. Look for prompt medical care if you, or someone you are with, **have symptoms of tremor.**

Note: hand tremor can also be due to low blood sugar, medications, mental health disorders, metabolic conditions, genetic disorders, and other abnormal processes. It can also occur with peripheral neuropathy as a complication of diabetes. In some instances, the cause of hand tremor is unknown.

Neurological Conditions

Some tremors are from problems in the deep parts of the brain that control movement. Some neurological conditions that can result in shaky hands include:

- **Multiple Sclerosis (MS)** - this degenerative disease will attack the brain and spinal cord, making it difficult for the nerves to relay messages. Many individuals with MS experience some degree of tremor, with it developing when the disease damages areas in the central nervous system's pathways that control movement.

Parkinson's disease (PD) - involves a loss of nerve cells in a part of the brain that performs a critical role in the motor movement. About 75% of people with PD have tremor, whether resting, action, or mixed. Tremor generally begins on one side of the body and spreads to the opposite side. Shaking can become more pronounced during periods of stress or strong emotion.

- **Parkinsonian tremor** - is caused by brain changes leading to abnormal movement. People with Parkinson's disease experience rigidity of the arms, legs, and trunk and eventually develop bradykinesia, a sluggish movement that includes the abrupt freezing of muscle movement. They can also have problems with balance and coordination. The exact cause of Parkinson's disease is unknown, but research suggests that genetic and environmental factors play a role.

- **Stroke** - after a stroke, an individual can have multiple tremors depending on the area affected. Damage to the basal ganglia causes **resting tremor,** while damage to the cerebellum causes **intentional tremor.**

- **Traumatic brain injury (TBI)** - a consequence of TBI is called **post-traumatic tremor (PTT).** This can happen due to damage to specific brain areas responsible for movement. This tremor is uncommon.

- **Dystonia** - a motion disorder in which involuntary muscle contractions cause repetitive, involuntary movements and postures. The condition is due to the brain's improper basal ganglia functioning. Tremor occurring in people with dystonia are either jerky and irregular, regular and wave-like, or mixed. Mixed types commonly affect the hands.

Hand Tremor Conditions and Symptoms

General Health Conditions
The following health conditions can cause shaky hands:

- Alcohol misuse or withdrawal
- Anxiety or panic
- Hyperthyroidism
- Inherited degenerative disorders, like hereditary ataxia or fragile X syndrome
- Liver or kidney failure
- Mercury poisoning
- Psychiatric conditions, like depression or post-traumatic stress disorder (PTT)

Symptoms That Might Occur With Hand Tremor
Hand tremor may occur with other symptoms, depending on the underlying disease, disorder, or condition. These symptoms can be characteristic of various ailments, including essential tremors, stroke, or hyperthyroidism.

Symptoms to be aware of:

- Frequent urination
- Impaired balance and coordination
- Numbness or tingling in any part of the body
- Quavering voice
- Shuffling gait (walk)
- Signs of hyperthyroidism, such as protruding eyes, unexplained weight loss, heat intolerance, perspiration, and goiter
- Signs of Multiple Sclerosis, such as weakness, numbness or tingling, vision problems, unsteady walk, fatigue, and depression

- Stooped posture
- Symptoms that might indicate a life-threatening condition

In some cases, hand tremor could occur with other indicators that could indicate a significant or life-threatening illness, such as a stroke, which can be evaluated in the Emergency Room. Immediately seek medical care (call 911) if you, or someone you are with, has any life-threatening symptoms such as:

- Confusion or loss of consciousness for a moment
- Difficulty breathing
- Difficulty speaking or understanding speech
- Difficulty walking
- Head injury
- Loss of vision or changes in vision
- Paralysis
- Rapid, involuntary rolling of the eyes (nystagmus)
- Rigid trunk
- Slurred speech
- Tremor on one side of the body
- Weakness (loss of strength)

SECTION 3 CAUSES of HAND TREMOR

Not Always a Disease

Shaky hands do not always indicate an illness. Sometimes tremor is the body's response to a condition such as:

- **B12 Deficiency** - the nervous system will not work like it should without it. You can find B12 in meat, fish, poultry, eggs, and milk products. It keeps your nervous system healthy.

- **Caffeine** - coffee may cause the hands to shake because it is a stimulant. The same natural chemical that helps you wake up will also make your hands shake if you have too much. You can find caffeine in over-the-counter headache medicine, chocolate, and some sodas.

- **Drugs** - a most common culprit is a medication that blocks a brain chemical called dopamine. It moves information from one part of the brain to another. These drugs are utilized to keep your mood even.

- **Low blood sugar** - called hypoglycemia, it triggers the body's natural stress response and makes you shaky.

- **Nerve damage** - injury, disease, or a problem with your central nervous system can also cause tremor. Your doctor will call this peripheral neuropathy. It can affect your hands and feet.

- **Overactive thyroid** - this gland is in your neck, just above your collarbone. When in overdrive, the entire body speeds up. You may have difficulty sleeping, your heart may beat faster, and your hands shake.

- **Sleep** - when you do not get enough sleep, it can cause your brain to tell your hands to tremble mistakenly. Here, you can snooze your way back to steady hands.

- **Smoking** - a significant cause of anxiety. Nicotine, the most addictive drug in tobacco, gets into your bloodstream and makes your heartbeat faster. It makes you feel anxious and can cause your hands to shake.

- **Stress** - worsens tremor and can make hands shake. Stress is known as **physiologic tremor.**

Since the causes and treatments vary widely for different tremors, talking with your doctor about your history and symptoms is essential.

Potential Causes Of Hand Tremor

Hand tremor originates in many diseases, disorders, and conditions, including:

- Alcoholism and alcohol withdrawal
- Brain damage from a stroke or tumor
- Essential tremor
- Extreme emotion, anxiety, or stress
- Hyperthyroidism
- Low blood sugar (hypoglycemia)
- Movement disorder (dystonia)
- Multiple sclerosis
- Nerve damage (peripheral neuropathy)
- Parkinson's disease
- Physical exhaustion
- Psychological disorder

Potential Medications That Cause Tremor Symptoms

Medications and drug withdrawals that can generate tremor symptoms include:

- Amiodarone (used to treat ventricular arrhythmia)
- Antidepressants and mood stabilizers
- Antiseizure medication
- Benzodiazepine withdrawal
- Bronchodilators
- Lithium
- Pseudoephedrine
- Theophylline

Certain drugs can cause hand tremor. Examples include:

- Amphetamine
- Anti-arrhythmic drugs, such as procainamide
- Caffeine
- Cancer medications, such as thalidomide
- Certain antiviral drugs
- Corticosteroids
- Medications that suppress the immune system, such as cyclosporine
- Seizure medications, such as valproate (Depakene) and valproic acid (Depakote)
- Some asthma medications
- Specific antibiotics

Medications and substances that may exacerbate tremor include:

- Atorvastatin (Lipitor)
- Beta-adrenergic agonists (e.g., albuterol)
- Carbamazepine (Tegretol)
- Cyclosporine (Sandimmune)
- Epinephrine
- Fluoxetine (Prozac)
- Haloperidol
- Hypoglycemic agents
- Methylphenidate (Ritalin)
- Metoclopramide (Reglan)

- Second-generation antipsychotics
- Terbutaline
- Thyroid hormones
- Tricyclic antidepressants
- Valproic acid (Depakene)
- Verapamil

Complications Of Hand Tremor

Hand tremor is not due to a significant or life-threatening condition. But, the humiliation associated with a hand tremor can be debilitating. Because hand tremor can be caused by critical illness, failure to seek treatment can result in complications. It is crucial to see your doctor when you experience tremor without an apparent cause.

Once the underlying cause is diagnosed, in following the treatment plan outlined by your doctor, you can lower the risk of potential complications, including:

- Difficulty performing daily tasks
- Embarrassment
- Impaired coordination
- Withdrawal or depression

Hand Tremor Triggers

If you have experienced hand tremor, you should look at some of the causes listed below and make some minor adjustments to your lifestyle to see if this makes a difference to your condition. If your disorder remains unchanged or becomes any worse, then you should make an appointment with your doctor to find its root cause.

The following are hand tremor triggers to be aware of:

Caffeine Toxicity
People state that they cannot start their day without a cup or two of coffee. Eventually, these people will find that they rely on coffee to get them through the morning the afternoon and soon drink eight, twelve, or more cups a day.

They might even switch directly from drinking coffee to something much more robust like energy drinks or caffeine tablets. This consumption can have many side effects, including heart palpitations and chest pain. You could also be putting yourself in danger of cardiac arrest if you have consumed too much caffeine, especially if you already have an underlying heart problem.
Note: hand tremor are common when you are suffering from caffeine toxicity, and most often, switching to decaf is enough to make the tremor disappear.

Pinched Nerve
If experiencing a tremor and you cannot find the cause, you may have a pinched nerve, especially if it is only occurring in one hand. A few other symptoms that tend to go along with a

pinched nerve include tingling or numbness in the elbows or fingertips: This could be a possible pinched nerve in your neck, back, shoulder, or elbow, sometimes even in your wrist.

Nerve Regen

The best course of action if you suspect that a pinched nerve is behind the tremor is to see your doctor for professional help. During the interim period, apply a heat compress to the area to alleviate the symptoms of discomfort and pain you might experience. You might want to combine this with anti-inflammatory medication to reduce pain and swelling. Remember that you should never pick up anything heavy if you suspect a pinched nerve.

Medication Side-Effects

If you are experiencing sudden tremor when you have never had any problems before, you should question yourself about any new medications that you may have taken. It is common for a doctor to ask you this question when you present them with a list of symptoms.

Medications can often have plenty of contraindications that clash with conditions or medications you are taking, and they might provide you with a range of side effects. If you suspect it might be a medication causing your tremor, you should first read the medicine's inner leaflet and look for the contraindications and side-effects section.

The second step is to get in touch with your doctor. They should find the root cause of the tremor and recommend another medication that will not cause these contraindications or side effects.

Note: never stop taking your medications without contacting your doctor.

Underlying Heart Problems
If you are experiencing a tremor along with heart palpitations or chest pain, then it could be possible that you may have an underlying heart problem that needs addressing. Often, tremor can be triggered by heart problems, such as Barlow's syndrome, a precursor to a heart attack, angina, or impending heart failure. Heart palpitations are a common heart issue accompanying tremor.

Take note of changes in your health and make an appointment with your physician or cardiologist if you feel you might have a heart problem. Cardiac problems must be routinely watched, and you should have a doctor's appointment at least once every six months. Make a comprehensive list of the symptoms you are experiencing and discuss this with your doctor to be diagnosed and subsequently treated.

Parkinson's Disease
Parkinson's Disease is a neuron condition, which means that it is a condition that directly affects the brain. Tremor is one of the most common symptoms associated with Parkinson's disease. However, the disease has many other symptoms, including depression, mood swings, changes in appetite, and a very common gait associated with Parkinson's disease in the later stages.

Stress
If you have experienced a tremor and can link it to a general feeling of despair, doom, fear, or anxiety, then your tremor could easily be due to a stress condition. Shaking and tremor are

common symptoms of people undergoing a panic attack, which eventually calms down as the panic attack stops.

If stress is the reason behind your tremor, you should teach yourself some easy, natural techniques, including breathing, that can help your heart calm down until the tremor subsides. If you find that this is not enough, you should make an appointment with your doctor. Many medications can make panic attacks easier to manage.

Alcoholism

This can cause tremor, especially if the person in question starts to withdraw from alcohol. The tremor might subside with a moderate drink in this situation. It can be risky for a severe alcoholic to stop the drug on their own (or go cold turkey as it is commonly referred to).

Alcoholics experiencing a tremor will most likely be in the throes of withdrawal and should seek medical attention for the tremor to subside. Such tremor can be caused by nerve damage, and if the person has been drinking for a significant part of their life, they might have done permanent damage to their organs or nerves in the process. This could cause their tremor, which might not go away in such a severe condition. Treatment needs to be reviewed if you are struggling with alcoholism.

Stroke

Tremor can occur due to damage caused by a stroke. Here, the tremor and numbness will go away with rehabilitative treatment, depending on the severity of the stroke after several months or years. Other times the tremor can only be reduced and treated symptomatically.

Tremor can also happen as a warning sign that a stroke is about to occur. Other symptoms accompanying a stroke include numbness, trouble talking, and passing out.

Blood Sugar

Test your blood sugar regularly, especially if you have anyone in your immediate family who has had issues with their blood sugar or problems with their heart. You should also pay attention if you are overweight or if anyone in your family has diabetes. If your blood sugar drops due to any reason, then you will experience a range of symptoms that can include blurred vision, and you might even faint.

The key to raising your blood sugar in a hurry is ingesting salt. If you are having problems with your blood sugar dropping too low throughout the day, learn to have healthy snacks, keeping your blood sugar levels at a healthy baseline to ensure that you have fewer problems with the symptoms of tremor.

Shock

This can sometimes be the cause of **behindhand tremor**. The body experiences shock when it goes through an experience that overloads its responses. For instance, something physically or mentally traumatic, such as surgery or an accident. After surgery, people usually are given medication to alleviate shock, and shock is the reason why you might wake up shaking after having undergone surgery. It is also why people are told to eat right after surgery and before the hospital discharges them.

Shock is usually a combination of blood pressure, blood sugar, and heart rate dropping rapidly. The symptoms caused by shock can include tremor of the hands and body. Although, things like blurred vision, heart palpitations, and fainting spells can occur.

Diabetes

Hypoglycemia
If you are on diabetic medications, you are at risk of becoming hypoglycemic. Experiencing shakiness, such as hand tremor, may indicate hypoglycemia. When blood sugar falls below a safe level, this can occur. Glucose in the blood below 70 mg/dl is considered hypoglycemic and requires treatment at once. Additional symptoms of hypoglycemia include fatigue, confusion, hunger, sweating, and dizziness.

Diabetic Neuropathy
Diabetic neuropathy may occur because of chronically high blood sugar or hyperglycemia. Diabetic neuropathy is characterized as degeneration of nerve fibers from a reduction in blood flow and high blood glucose. Hand tremor may be a symptom of diabetic neuropathy, which indicates a problem with the nervous system. The trauma-affected nerves can result in the involuntary movements of a hand tremor. Keeping blood glucose under control and in a safe range can reduce the risk of developing neuropathy.

SECTION 4   TREATMENT

Seeking Medical Help

Typically, help for tremors can be obtained by visiting a Neurologist, a specialist in dealing with nervous system disorders. This specialist deals with diagnosing and treating all the conditions and diseases involving the central and peripheral nervous systems, including their coverings, blood vessels, and all effector tissue, such as muscle.

Questions The Doctor Will Ask

Your doctor will ask you questions about your symptoms to diagnose the underlying condition. Supplying detailed answers to these questions will help your doctor diagnose the cause of your hand tremor:

- How long have you had tremors?
- Do you have a family history of tremors?
- What medications are you taking (including nonprescription drugs and supplements)?
- What makes your hand tremor better or worse?
- Have you ever had a head injury?

Some Treatment Medications

What Medications Treat Shaky Hands?
Not everybody with shaky hands will need treatment. But, if your doctor determines that you are a candidate, they may prescribe medication.

Commonly Prescribed Medications
The **National Tremor Foundation** states that the most prescribed medications for treating shaky hands due to **essential tremor** are:

1) Antiseizure medications
   a) Primidone

2) Propranolol a beta-blocker designed to treat:
   a) arrhythmia
   b) fast heart rate
   c) hypertension

If the above medications do not work, your doctor may recommend other drugs such as:

- **Beta-blockers** - Metoprolol (Lopressor) and atenolol (Tenormin) are used to treat **essential tremors.** Your doctor might prescribe one of these medications if other medications do not help, but they may not work as well as propranolol.

- **Antiseizure medications** - Gabapentin (Neurontin) and topiramate (Topamax) are used to treat neurological or psychiatric conditions, like seizures or neuropathic pain. They can be helpful for people with **essential tremors.**

- **Anti-anxiety medication** - Alprazolam (Xanax) is used to treat anxiety (which can cause shaking hands) and panic disorders. However, research indicates that it might be an effective treatment for **essential tremors.** Take this drug with caution because it is habit-forming.

- **Botox** (Botulinum toxin type A) - shows promise as a treatment for **essential tremor** that affects the hands. This medicine may cause significant muscle weakness where injected, so be sure to speak with your doctor about the risks and benefits. Benefits from the injection can last up to 3 months, and then ensuing injections will be necessary.

Therapies and Surgery

Therapy

Doctors could suggest physical or occupational therapy, where:

Physical Therapists - may teach exercises to improve muscle strength, control, and coordination.

Occupational Therapists - may help you adapt to living with **essential tremors.** The therapists might suggest adaptive devices to reduce the effect of tremors on your daily activities, including:

- Broader, heavier writing tools, such as wide-grip pens
- Heavier glasses and utensils
- Wrist weights

Surgery

Some patients may experience a severe tremor that does not respond to medications or significantly impacts their life quality. In these cases, the doctor may recommend surgical interventions, such as **Deep Brain Stimulation (DBS).** Doctors use DBS to help treat tremor associated with **essential tremors, PD, or dystonia.**

- **Deep brain stimulation** - is the most common type of surgery for **essential tremors.** It is usually preferred by medical centers with significant experience in performing DBS.

- **Focused ultrasound thalamotomy** - is a non-invasive surgery involving focused sound waves that travel through skin and skull. The waves generate heat to destroy brain tissues in the specific thalamus area to stop the tremor. Surgeons use magnetic resonance imaging to target the precise location in the brain and ensure the sound waves generate the exact amount of heat needed for the procedure.

Focused ultrasound thalamotomy generates a lesion that can permanently change brain function. Some people have experienced the altered sensation, trouble walking, and movement. Still, most complications go away on their own or are mild enough not to interfere with life quality.

If an individual is not eligible for DBS, a doctor may recommend other procedures, such as:

- **Radiofrequency ablation** - involves using an electric current to heat nerve tissue to disrupt its ability to relay signals for several months.

- **Radiosurgery** - involves administering highly focused radiation beams to destroy the overactive brain cells causing the tremor.

Lifestyle Changes

Stop Hands From Shaking

Handshaking can hinder day-to-day living and quality of life, but there are ways to control it. Handshaking may be mild, moderate, or severe, but slight hand tremor is often caused by lifestyle choices that can be reduced through simple changes.

If you are suffering from severe hand tremor, see your doctor to diagnose and review your options because these are more often a symptom of a medical issue. It can be challenging to hold a cup in some extreme cases. Medication, therapy, or surgery may help calm shaking hands!

The following are some methods to employ to help stop hands from shaking:

- **Lifestyle changes** - the following lifestyle changes may help to reduce hand tremor in people with **enhanced physiologic tremor:**
  - get at least 7-hours of sleep to prevent tremor.
  - eat foods rich in vitamin B1
  - practice stress-fighting activities
  - avoiding vigorous exercise
  - avoiding excess alcohol consumption
  - avoiding stimulants, such as caffeine and amphetamines

- **Treating underlying conditions** - hand tremor that occurs because of an underlying condition, such as hyperthyroidism or alcohol withdrawal, typically improves following treatment for the underlying condition.

- **Psychological techniques** - people experiencing tremor because of anxiety or panic attacks can benefit from practicing relaxation techniques, like mindfulness and breathing exercises.

- **Switching medications** - tremor can be a side effect of taking certain drugs. A person who experiences tremor while taking medication should report the side effect to their doctor. The doctor can adjust the medication dosage or switch to a different drug.

- **Physical therapy** - the physical therapist can teach people exercises to improve the following:
  - muscle control, functioning, and strength
  - coordination
  - balance

- **Occupational therapy** - an occupational therapist can help people living with tremor continue engaging in their usual daily activities.

APPENDIX A - DISEASES, DISORDERS, & CONDITIONS

Fragile X Tremor Ataxias Syndrome (FXTAS)

This is an adult-onset neurodegenerative disorder, usually affecting males over 50 and females who comprise only a small part of the FXTAS population. Their symptoms are less severe than males. FXTAS affects the neurological systems and progresses at varying rates in different individuals.

Major FXTAS Symptoms include:

- **Gait ataxias** - balance problems which may include falling, needed support when walking or going up and downstairs, trouble stepping on/off curbs, generalized instability, or display of a wide-based gait.

- **Intention tremor** - a tremor of the hand when using utensils, writing instruments, reaching for, or pouring something.

- **MRI findings** - strongly associated with (but not unique to) FXTAS. These findings include white matter lesions involving signs of middle cerebellar peduncles (MCP).

- **Neuropathology** - findings called "FXTAS inclusions" within brain cells.

Minor FXTAS Symptoms include:

- **MRI** - findings that are more general than those listed above.

- **Parkinsonism** - (resting tremors).

- **Cognitive Problems** - with executive function and decision-making. Executive function allows us to solve problems and generalize from one situation to another.

- **Short-term memory problem**s - can be challenging to determine since it is natural for short-term memory to deteriorate as we age. However, FXTAS can change more rapidly than usual or even more dramatically. This includes forgetting what one ate, said, or did shortly after the event.

Hyperthyroidism (overactive thyroid)

Shaky hands may be a sign of hyperthyroidism. This means the thyroid gland is working too hard and kicking the heart rate into overdrive. You may also find that you will lose weight without trying, be sensitive to light, have a fast heartbeat, and have trouble sleeping. A blood test will help you and your doctor figure out what is happening.

Multiple Sclerosis (MS)

A disabling disease of the brain and spinal cord (central nervous system). With MS, the body's immune system attacks the protective sheath (myelin) that covers the nerve fibers causing transmission problems between the brain and the rest of the body. Finally, the disease can cause permanent damage or deterioration of the nerves.

Signs and symptoms of MS vary significantly and depend on the amount of nerve damage and which nerves are affected. Some individuals with severe MS can lose the ability to walk independently or at all, while others could experience long periods of remission without any new symptoms.

At this time, there is no cure for MS. But, treatments can help with recovery from attacks, modify the course of the disease, and manage its symptoms.

Multiple System Atrophy (MSA)

It is a progressive neurodegenerative disorder characterized by symptoms that affect the autonomic nervous system (controls involuntary actions such as blood pressure or digestion) and movement. Indicators reveal the progressive loss of function and the death of different nerve cells in the brain and spinal cord.

Indicators of autonomic failure found in MSA include fainting spells, heart rate problems, erectile dysfunction, and bladder control. Motor impairments (lost or limited muscle control, movement, or limited mobility) may include tremor, rigidity, muscle coordination loss, as well as difficulties with speech and gait (the way a person walks). Some of these features are similar to those in Parkinson's disease.

MSA is a rare disease with symptoms that tend to appear in a person in their 50s, and it advances rapidly over 5 to 10 years, with progressive loss of motor function and eventual confinement to bed. Individuals with MSA often develop pneumonia in the later stages of the disease and may suddenly die from cardiac or respiratory issues.

Neurodegenerative Disease

These diseases happen when nerve cells in the brain or the peripheral nervous system lose function with time and ultimately die. Although treatment may help alleviate some of the physical or mental symptoms associated with the diseases, there is no way to slow disease progression, and there are no known cures.

The risks of being affected by a neurodegenerative disease increase dramatically with age. With people living longer lives today, more people may be affected by neurodegenerative diseases.

Parkinson's Disease (PD)

Parkinson's disease is a progressive nervous system disorder that affects movement. Symptoms start gradually, sometimes with a barely noticeable tremor in just one hand. Tremors are typical, but the disease also commonly causes stiffness or slowing of movement.

Although Parkinson's disease cannot be cured, medications can significantly improve symptoms. Your doctor may recommend surgery to regulate particular brain regions and improve your symptoms in specific situations.

Parkinson's signs and symptoms can be different for everyone. Early indications may be mild and go unnoticed. Indicators often start on one side of the body and usually remain harsher on that side, even after symptoms affect both sides.

Parkinson's signs and symptoms include:

- **Impaired posture and balance** - posture can become stooped, or you may have balance problems because of Parkinson's disease.

- **Loss of automatic movements** - you may have a decreased ability to perform unconscious actions, including blinking, smiling, or swinging your arms when you walk.

- **Rigid muscles** - stiff muscles may occur in any part of the body. The stiff muscles may be painful and limit the range of motion.

- **Slowed movement (bradykinesia)** - Parkinson's disease may slow activities over time, making simple tasks difficult and time-consuming, your stride may become shorter when you walk, it may be challenging getting up from a chair, and you may find yourself dragging your feet as you try to walk.

- **Speech changes** - you may speak softly, quickly, slur, or hesitate before talking. Your speech may be more monotone rather than the usual inflections.

- **Tremor** - a tremor or shaking, usually beginning in a limb, your hand, or your fingers. Here you may rub your thumb and forefinger back and forth, known as a pill-rolling tremor, and your hand may tremble when it is at rest.

- **Writing changes** - may become difficult to write, and characters may appear small.

Pheochromocytoma

A sporadic tumor that grows in your adrenal gland. Though the tumor is usually benign, it increases your blood pressure. It could make you shake and cause heavy sweating, shortness of breath, and headaches. The tumor may also lead to heart disease and stroke. It is best to remove the tumor with surgery.

Tardive Dyskinesia

It is a neurological disorder that makes it difficult for individuals to control their movements adequately and difficult to perform daily tasks. This disorder often occurs when a person takes antipsychotic medications for a while. Though antipsychotics are helpful for certain mental health conditions, their dopamine suppressing effect can cause some nervous system issues.

Wilson's Disease

Shaking is a symptom of some liver disorders, such as Wilson's disease. A buildup of copper in the body damages your liver and brain in its genetic condition. You will feel tired and get jaundice (a yellow tint to your eyes and skin). Doctors treat **Wilson's Disease** with medications and diet changes.

APPENDIX B - TREATMENTS & EQUIPMENT

Deep Brain Stimulation (DBS)

In DBS surgery, an electrode is inserted into the targeted area of the brain (thalamus), causing the tremor, using MRI (magnetic resonance imaging) and recording the brain cell activity during the procedure. Subsequently, a second procedure is performed, implanting a pacemaker-like device (neurostimulator) in the chest. A wire travels under the skin connecting this device to the electrodes in your brain. The device transmits painless electrical pulses that interrupt signals from the thalamus that may be causing the tremor.

Like all brain surgeries, DBS carries a slight risk of infection, stroke, bleeding, or seizures. DBS surgery can be associated with reduced clarity of speech.

The Facts

- Surgical procedures treat various disabling neurological symptoms, most commonly the debilitating symptoms of Parkinson's, such as tremor, rigidity, stiffness, slowed movement, and walking.

- DBS surgery treats several conditions, such as **essential tremor**, dystonia, epilepsy, obsessive-compulsive disorder, and other common neurological movement disorders.

- DMS surgery does not damage healthy brain tissue or destroy nerve cells. On the other hand, the procedure interrupts problematic electrical signals from targeted areas in the brain.

- DMS uses a surgically implanted, battery-operated medical device called a neurostimulator (about the size of a stopwatch) to deliver electrical stimulation to the targeted areas in the brain that control movement by preventing abnormal nerve signals that cause the tremor and PD symptoms. Before the procedure, the neurosurgeon uses magnetic resonance imaging (MRI) or computed tomography (CT) to scan, identify, and locate the target in the brain where electrical nerve signals generate PD symptoms.

- During the surgery, some surgeons may use microelectrode recording, which involves a small wire that monitors the activity of nerve cells in the targeted area, identifying the precise brain target for stimulation. In general, the targets are the thalamus, subthalamic nucleus (STN), and a section of the globus pallidus.

- When the system is in place, electrical impulses from the neurostimulator go up along the extension wire and the active contacts of the lead in the brain. These impulses interfere with and block the electrical signals that cause PD symptoms.

The DBS System Consists of Three Components

- The lead (also called an electrode) is a thin, insulated wire inserted through a small opening in the skull and implanted in the brain. The tip of the electrode is placed within the affected area of the brain.

- The extension is an insulated wire that passes under the skin connecting the lead to the neurostimulator.

- The neurostimulator (battery pack) is the third component implanted near the collarbone's skin. In some cases, it might be implanted lower in the chest or under the skin over the abdomen.

The Prognosis
While most people will still need to take medication after undergoing DBS, many will experience a considerable reduction of their symptoms and dramatically reduce their medication. The amount of reduction can vary from person to person.

The reduction in medication leads to decreased risk of side effects such as dyskinesia (involuntary movements of the arms, legs, and head). There is a one to three percent chance of infection, stroke, cranial bleeding, or other complications associated with anesthesia, per side that is done. It is best to discuss associated risks with your neurologist and neurosurgeon.

Focused Ultrasound Thalamotomy

It is a non-invasive, therapeutic technology that can improve the quality of life and reduce the cost of care for patients suffering essential tremor. This novel technology uses multiple focused beams of ultrasound energy precisely and accurately targeted deep in the brain without damaging normal tissue.

How it Works
The focused ultrasound beams converge, producing precise ablation (thermal destruction of tissue), enabling **essential tremor** to be treated non-invasively. The target is a region in the thalamus called the ventral intermediate nucleus (Vim), but other adjacent targets and white matter pathways are also used.

Advantages

- It is a non-invasive, single treatment enabling patients to recover rapidly and return to normal life activities (usually the following day).

- Compared with RF ablation or DBS, focused ultrasound reduces infection risk, damage to the non-targeted area, and blood clot formation.

- Focused ultrasound offers a rapid resolution of symptoms.

- Focused ultrasound does not use ionizing radiation, thereby avoiding the side effects of radiation exposure.

- Because it is non-invasive, focused ultrasound could be an option for medically refractory ET patients who do not respond well to medication and do not want surgery.

FYI:

Focused ultrasound treatment for essential tremor received approved by the Food and Drug Administration (FDA) in July 2016.

Medicare-approved the treatment in all US states as of July 12, 2020.

Magnetic Resonance Imaging (MRI)

A non-invasive imaging technology that produces three-dimensional detailed anatomical images. It is frequently used for disease detection, diagnosis, and treatment monitoring. The technology is based on exciting and detecting changes in the rotational axis of protons found in the water that makes up living tissues.

The Risks

Even though MRI does not emit the ionizing radiation found in x-ray and CT imaging, it employs a powerful magnetic field. This field extends beyond the machine and exerts powerful forces on objects made of iron, some steel, and other magnetizable things. Patients should notify their physicians of any implant before an MRI scan.

When having an MRI scan, be aware of the following:

- **Claustrophobia** - people with claustrophobia may find it challenging to tolerate the long scan times inside the machine. Familiarization with the machine, process and visualization techniques, sedation, and anesthesia provide patients with methods to overcome their discomfort.
  - The open MRI is a machine open on the sides rather than a tube closed at one end, so it does not envelop the patient.

- **Contrast agents** - patients with diabetes that require dialysis may risk a rare but severe illness called Nephrogenic Systemic Fibrosis associated with the use of specific gadolinium-containing agents. Although a link has not been established, present guidelines in the

United States recommend that dialysis patients should only receive gadolinium agents when necessary and that dialysis must be completed after the scan to remove the agent from the patient's body.

- **Nerve Stimulation** - a twitching sensation occasionally results from the rapidly switched fields in the MRI.

- **Noise** - loud noise commonly called clicking and beeping, and sound intensity up to 120 decibels in specific MR scanners may require special ear protection.

- **People with implants** - that contain iron, pacemakers, vagus nerve stimulators, implantable cardioverter-defibrillators, loop recorders, insulin pumps, cochlear implants, deep brain stimulators, and capsules from capsule endoscopy must not enter an MRI machine.

- **Pregnancy** - while no effects have been identified in the fetus, MRI scans should be avoided as a precaution, especially during the first trimester of pregnancy when the fetus' organs are being formed and the contrast agents, if used, could enter the fetus's bloodstream.

Nerve Conduction Study (NCS)

What Is EMG (electromyogram)?
It is a test that evaluates electrical activity within the nerves and muscles. Your doctor might recommend getting an EMG to diagnose muscle weakness, muscular dystrophy, and other neuromuscular abnormalities. An EMG test entails inserting tiny needles into the muscles to record electrical activity and how well the muscles respond to those signals. If your test picks up a problem, you will be diagnosed with a **neuromuscular disorder.**

What Is NCS?
Nerve signals are electrical impulses that travel quickly throughout the nervous system. Sometimes, problems with electrical activity in the nerves can cause pain, tingling, or weakness. NCS measures how fast and how strong the electrical activity is in a nerve. The test can additionally tell if a nerve is damaged.

Do I Need EMG or NCS?
Your doctor will determine the tests you need after evaluating your condition.

Note: talk with your doctor about taking any medications before being evaluated. There may be some medications that you should avoid until after the test. If you have a pacemaker, tell your doctor before scheduling an NCS or EMG.

APPENDIX C - RESOURCES

Organizations

Focused Ultrasound Foundation 1230 Cedars Court, Ste 206 Charlottesville, VA 22903	(434) 220.4993 https://www.fusfoundation.org/diseases-and-conditions/neurological/essential-tremor
Mayo Clinic 5777 E. Mayo Blvd. Phoenix, AZ 85054 4500 San Pablo Road Jacksonville, FL 32224 200 First St. SW Rochester, MN 55905	General Number: (480) 301-8000 https://www.mayoclinic.org/
National Institute of Environmental Health Sciences (NIH) 111 Tw Alexander Dr # A2-09 Durham, NC 27709	(919) 541-4704 https://www.niehs.nih.gov/
National Institute of Neurological Disorders (NIH) 31 Center Dr Bethesda, MD 20892	(301) 496-5751 https://www.ninds.nih.gov/
Parkinson's Foundation 200 SE 1st Street, Ste 800 Miami, FL 33131, USA 1359 Broadway, Ste 1509 New York, NY 10018, USA	(800) 473-4636 https://www.parkinson.org/Understanding-Parkinsons/Treatment/Surgical-Treatment-Options/Deep-Brain-Stimulation
The National Fragile X Foundation 1861 International Drive, Ste. 200, McLean, VA 22102	(800) 688-8765 https://fragilex.org/understanding-fragile-x/tremor-ataxia-syndrome-fxtas/

Website Articles

Mayo Clinic	
Essential Tremor Written By Mayo Clinic Staff https://www.mayoclinic.org/diseases-conditions/essential-tremor/symptoms-causes/syc-20350534	
MedicalNewsToday	
Why are my hands shaking? Causes, is it normal, and remedies Written by Amanda Barrell - Updated on January 13, 2022 https://www.medicalnewstoday.com/articles/322195	
Very Healthy Life	
10 Hand Tremors Causes Everyone Should Be Aware Of https://veryhealthy.life/10-hand-tremors-causes-everyone-should-be-aware-of/?utm_source=%2Bhand%20%2Btremor&utm_medium=10HandTremorsCauses&utm_campaign=adw_us	
Verywell Health	
Radiofrequency Ablation: Everything You Need to Know https://www.verywellhealth.com/radiofrequency-ablation-5096619	
WebMD	
Reasons Your Hands Are Shaking https://www.webmd.com/parkinsons-disease/ss/slideshow-reasons-your-hands-are-shaking What is EMG and Nerve Conduction Study? https://www.webmd.com/brain/emg-and-nerve-conduction-study	

AFTERWORD

Thank you for reading,

TREMORS
What Is Hand Tremor
Signs, Symptoms, and Treatment

We hope you enjoyed this
Life-Health Media USA Publication

Thank you again, valued reader,
and we hope to meet you again on another book.

ABOUT THE AUTHOR

Pierre Mouchette is the Founder and CEO of Real Property Experts LLC. He is a graduate of New York University, with a Master's in Business Administration, a Certificate in Real Estate Law - Fairfield University - CT, a Graduate of the Realtors Institute - CT, and held licensing as a Real Estate Broker, and a Mortgage Broker.

Pierre is currently authoring Books, Booklets, How-to-Articles, and Guides in retirement. Pierre has an extensive background in real estate investment, business management, and sales, supplemented by decades of hands-on experience in building systems engineering, development, evaluation, and various analytical engineering studies.

Pierre launched Real Property Experts in 2013 to simplify real estate investing by connecting investors through innovative technology using background knowledge and experience. In 2018, Pierre created THE SYNCHRONICITY INVESTOR, a real estate website to facilitate world-class solutions for real estate investors and investment businesses.

Life-Health Media USA

- presents -

An Enviro | Life Knowledge Publications

LIFE HEALTH

HEALTH and DISEASES

MENIER'S DISEASE – What Is Meniere's, Symptoms, Treatment, and Lifestyle

OVERACTIVE BLADDER – Symptoms, Treatments, and Lifestyle Remedies

TREMORS - What Is Hand Tremor, Signs, Symptoms, and Treatment

www.ingramcontent.com/pod-product-compliance
Lightning Source LLC
Chambersburg PA
CBHW070125230526
45472CB00004B/1419